WAYS TO RAISE TESTOSTERONE LEVELS

COMPLETE GUIDE REGARDING TESTOSTERONE

HERB LAWRENCE

2

Contents

chapter 1

WHAT EFFECTS DO HORMONES HAVE ON A MAN'S BODY12

chapter 2

PELLETS OF TESTOSTERONE

chapter 3

HYPOGONADISM

chapter 4

AGE RELATED CHANGES IN TESTOSTERONE

chapter 5

METHODS THAT HAVE BEEN PROVEN TO BOOST TESTOSTERONE NATURALLY

chapter 6

FOODS THAT ARE LOW IN TESTOSTERONE

Chapter 7

TESTOSTERONE BOOSTING SUPPLEMENTS

chapter 8

THE EFFECTS OF ALCOHOL ON TESTOSTERONE

chapter 1

THE ROLE OF HORMONES IN MEN

To produce sperm, testosterone stimulates the activity of cells in the testicles. Overall health depends on testosterone levels as well. Bone health is improved, and one's disposition and libido are influenced as a result. The conversion of some testosterone into estrogen, the female sex hormone, is necessary for bone health.

To put it simply, hormones are crucial to the male reproductive system. They influence a man's fertility and are ultimately accountable for sex urges.

WHAT EFFECTS DO HORMONES HAVE ON A MAN'S BODY

One of the most vital hormones is testosterone. It has been shown to improve libido, muscle mass, memory, and energy levels. But as men age, their testosterone levels naturally drop. Between 20% and 40% of males over the age of 40 suffer from hypogonadism, a medical disease treated by using testosterone replacement medication.

A LOOK AT TESTOSTERONE'S REPERCUSSIONS FOR THE HUMAN BODY

For men, testosterone is a crucial hormone. In a male, testosterone production can start as early as seven weeks after conception. During puberty, testosterone levels increase, peak in the late teenage years, and then stabilize. The testosterone levels of men naturally decline at a slow but steady rate beyond the age of 30.

In most cases, guys have plenty of testosterone. However, low testosterone levels can occur in men. Hypogonadism is the ensuing medical condition. Hormone replacement treatment, which must be prescribed by a doctor and closely monitored, can help. When testosterone levels are normal, a man should not take testosterone supplements.

Men's testosterone levels have far-reaching effects, influencing everything from reproductive health and sexual drive to physical strength and bone density. Additionally, it influences some actions.

A LOOK AT THE ENDOCRINE SYSTEM

Hormones are produced by the glands that make up the endocrine system. The pituitary gland receives instructions about how much testosterone to produce from the hypothalamus in the brain. After receiving the signal, the pituitary gland relays it to the male reproductive organs. Though the testicles are responsible for producing the vast majority of testosterone, the adrenal glands, which sit above the kidneys, also contribute a minor quantity. Low levels of testosterone are made by the adrenal glands and ovaries in females.

Testosterone plays a role in the development of male genitalia before a guy is even born. At puberty, testosterone causes the growth of male characteristics such a deeper voice, beard, and body hair. The development of muscle and the arousal to engage in sexual activity are two more benefits. Adolescence is marked by a dramatic increase in testosterone production, which reaches its peak in one's late teens or early 20s. Approximately 1% of testosterone is lost every year after age 30.

THE PHYSIOLOGY OF REPRODUCTION

Testosterone plays a role in shaping the male genitalia beginning about week seven of pregnancy. The testicles and penis enlarge during puberty as a result of an increase in testosterone production. Daily, the testicles create new sperm and a fresh stream of testosterone.

Erectile dysfunction has been linked to decreased testosterone levels in men (ED). Chronic testosterone replacement medication has been linked to a drop in sperm count. In addition to an enlarged prostate, testosterone therapy has been linked to testicular atrophy and decreased virility. In males who have had either prostate or breast cancer, the use of testosterone replacement treatment is not recommended.

SEXUALITY

Testicles, penis, and pubic hair develop in response to increasing levels of testosterone during adolescence. Muscles and hair start to sprout, and a deeper voice emerges. Increased sexual desire is a natural consequence of these alterations.

The old adage "use it or lose it" isn't completely false. If a man's testosterone levels are low, he may lose interest in having sexual relations with other men. Both sexual interest and activity raise testosterone levels. When a man is sexually inactive for an extended period, his testosterone levels can drop. Similarly to low estrogen, low testosterone can cause erectile dysfunction (ED).

ANATOMY OF THE BRAIN AND SPINAL CORD

The body has a system for managing testosterone, sending messages through hormones and chemicals that are released into the bloodstream. The testicles receive their instructions for producing testosterone from the pituitary gland, which in turn receives them from the hypothalamus in the brain.

Aggression and a desire to be dominant are two of the behaviors that may be influenced by testosterone. It also encourages healthy competition and improves confidence. Participating in competitive activities can increase or decrease a man's testosterone levels, just as sexual activity might. Having low testosterone levels can make you feel down on yourself and uninspired. It might also make a man unhappy or affect his concentration. Reduced testosterone levels are associated with fatigue and disturbed sleep.

It's crucial to highlight, however, that testosterone is simply one component that determines personality traits. There are undoubtedly more biological and environmental elements at play.

FOLLICLES AND SCALP

As a man goes from childhood to maturity, testosterone encourages the growth of hair on the face, in the armpits, and around the genitals. The arms, legs, and chest are not immune to hair growth.

A man with declining levels of testosterone truly may lose some body hair. Testosterone replacement medication comes with a few potential side effects, including acne and breast growth. Testosterone patches may cause slight skin discomfort. Topical gels may be easier to use, but great caution must be taken to avoid spreading testosterone to someone else by skin-to-skin contact.

THERE'S MUSCLE, FAT, AND BONE

Involvement of testosterone in the process of gaining muscle mass and strength is just one of many. Testosterone raises levels of neurotransmitters that stimulate tissue expansion. It also triggers protein synthesis by interacting with DNA nuclear receptors. The levels of growth hormone are raised by testosterone. That's why working out is so effective for muscle gain.

Testosterone enhances bone density and tells the bone marrow to generate red blood cells. Men with very low levels of testosterone are more likely to suffer from bone fractures and breaks.

Testosterone also aids fat metabolism, making it easier for men to lose weight. Body fat increases with declining testostcrone levels.

Injections of testosterone into the muscle tissue by a medical professional is one method of delivering the hormone for testosterone replacement therapy.

SYSTEM OF THE HEART AND BLOOD VESSELS

As a hormone, testosterone circulates throughout the body. Your testosterone level can only be determined with certainty by having it measured. A blood test is typically needed for this.

The production of red blood cells is stimulated by testosterone in the bone marrow. And there is evidence from research that testosterone might even be good for the cardiovascular system. However, there has been conflicting evidence from research looking at testosterone's impact on lipids, hypertension, and blood clotting.

Recent investigations on the effects of testosterone therapy on the cardiovascular system have yielded inconsistent results, and this research is still under progress. High blood cell counts may result from intramuscular testosterone injectable therapy. Fluid retention, an elevated red cell count, and alterations to cholesterol levels are additional negative effects of testosterone replacement treatment.

TESTOSTERONE HOW DOES IT WORK

Testosterone levels in men are strictly regulated to keep them at a healthy range, and while they tend to be highest in the morning and drop during the day, they never get too high. Key regulators of testicular testosterone production include the hypothalamus and pituitary gland. As a result of the hypothalamus secreting gonadotrophin-releasing hormone, the pituitary gland generates luteinizing hormone, which then enters the bloodstream and stimulates the gonads to make and release testosterone.

There is a negative feedback loop whereby elevated testosterone levels in the blood reduce the hypothalamic release of gonadotrophin-releasing hormone, which in turn reduces pituitary synthesis of luteinizing hormone. As a result, testosterone levels drop, negative feedback weakens, and the hypothalamus once again secretes gonadotrophin-releasing hormone.

WHAT WOULD HAPPEN IF MY TESTOSTERONE LEVELS WERE EXCESSIVE

The physiological effects of elevated testosterone levels vary with age and sex. Too much testosterone is difficult to detect in adult males since it is unusual that men will acquire a disease that causes them to create too much testosterone. More plainly, too much testosterone can cause aberrant genital development in young girls and a false growth spurt in young toddlers. Premature puberty and infertility are two of the many negative outcomes of elevated testosterone levels, which can affect both sexes.

One possible sign of polycystic ovarian syndrome in women is elevated testosterone levels in the blood. Acne, body and facial hair (called hirsutism), hair loss at the crown, bulking up, and a deeper voice are all possible side effects of this illness in women.

Excessive levels of testosterone can also be caused by a number of medical disorders. Androgen resistance, adrenal hyperplasia in infants, and ovarian cancer are all in this category.

In men, the production of testosterone and sperm in the testes is reduced while they are on anabolic steroids (made androgenic hormones) because the pituitary gland's secretion of luteinizing hormone and follicle stimulating hormone is suppressed. Anabolic steroids have been linked to a number of negative health effects in men, including reduced libido, a thinning of the testicles, and the development of breast tissue. Overworking the liver to eliminate the anabolic steroids could lead to serious health problems. Alterations in behavior (such heightened irritation) could also surface. As a high concentration of testosterone, whether natural or synthetic, can promote masculinization (virilization), anabolic steroids also create undesirable effects in women who take them consistently.

WHAT WOULD HAPPEN IF MY TESTOSTERONE LEVELS WERE TOO LOW

Fetal testosterone shortage can prevent the full maturation of masculine traits. A lack of testosterone during puberty might cause a boy's growth to halt, and he might not have a typical growth spurt. Changes in the child's vocal pitch, the growth of pubic hair, and the size of the penis and testes may be slowed. Boys with low testosterone levels may experience a delay in puberty, a loss of muscle mass, and continued disproportionate growth of the arms and legs.

Low testosterone levels in males of reproductive age have been linked to a loss of muscle mass, balding, and a wrinkly, "parchment-like" appearance of the skin. Testosterone levels naturally decrease in males as they become older. In the media, this is sometimes referred to as the male menopause (andropause) (andropause).

Low testosterone levels have been linked to mood disorders, weight gain, muscle loss, poor erections and performance in the bedroom, bone fragility, memory loss, trouble focusing, and disturbed sleep. Current research reveals that this impact happens in only a minority (approximately 2%) of ageing men. Lots of studies are presently being conducted to learn more about testosterone's effects in older men and the potential benefits of testosterone replacement treatment.

chapter 2

PELLETS OF TESTOSTERONE

After having testosterone pellets implanted, a patient may feel more energized, sleep better, and have an overall better quality of life. Gains in muscle and bone density are possible, along with a reduction in body fat. Strength, coordination, and physical performance may all improve for some patients.

LEARN ABOUT TESTOSTERONE

One of the most vital hormones is testosterone. It has been shown to improve libido, muscle mass, memory, and energy levels. But as men age, their testosterone levels naturally drop.

A reported 20 to 40 percent of elderly men have a medical issue termed hypogonadism and need testosterone replacement treatment (TRT). But there are downsides to TRT, including the chance for heart disease, excessive red blood cell count, and other disorders.

Getting the proper dose of the right hormone therapy delivery mechanism is crucial for a positive outcome. You can get patches, lotions, injections, or even pellets of testosterone.

Pellets may be an excellent option for those desiring a steady, long-term dose. You and your doctor can have a conversation about the many treatment strategies available to you.

PELLETS OF TESTOSTERONE

A tiny pellet of testosterone, like Test Opel, is available. They contain crystalline testosterone and measure 3 mm by 9 mm. They're implanted under the skin and gradually deliver testosterone over the period of three to six months.

The pellets are implanted subcutaneously, typically near the hip, during a quick and easy surgery performed in your doctor's office.

A long-lasting kind of testosterone replacement therapy, these pellets last for a whole year. They need to provide a constant stream of testosterone, usually enough to last for four months.

DIAGNOSING THE OPTIMAL DOSE

It may take a while to find the optimal dose that effectively treats your low testosterone symptoms. Dangerous side effects, such as an increase in red blood cell count, can be brought on by an excess of testosterone (RBC). According to studies, there are additional dangers associated with high testosterone levels.

Some people may have trouble determining an appropriate dosage. It is possible to identify the optimal dose for your body by working with your doctor, who may also be able to guide you toward the optimal treatment strategy.

TESTOSTERONE DOSING: THE HIGHS AND LOWS

Easy-to-self-administer topical treatments like creams, gels, buccal tablets, nasal spray (nates to), underarm solution (axion), and patches require regular application.

You also run the danger of mistakenly exposing women and infants to contact with excessive quantities of testosterone.

Injections have the potential to persist longer and avoid the contact issues of the aforementioned approaches. Still, injection-site discomfort is a possibility. You have to go to a healthcare provider or learn to inject yourself.

Some of the unpleasant side effects of TRT are attributable to the highs and lows of testosterone dose with conventional administration methods.

Testosterone levels, after being artificially boosted with injections, can fluctuate widely between very high and very low. There may be a dramatic swing in mood, libido, and energy levels as a result.

Estrogens like estradiol are produced when testosterone is broken down at its maximal levels of exposure. This much estrogen can potentially contribute to breast development and pain.

TRT MAY ALSO CAUSE THE FOLLOWING UNWANTED EFFECTS

sleep apnea

acne

low sperm count

larger than average breasts

testicular atrophy

enhanced RBC

Placement of Pellet Implants

The average time for an implant surgery is around 10 minutes.

After scrubbing the upper hip or buttocks area, a local anesthetic is given under the skin to dull any pain. A tiny incision is made.

With the help of a trocar, little pellets of testosterone are inserted under the skin. In most cases, ten to twelve pellets will be implanted. After around 4 months, you'll need to repeat the process because the effects have worn off.

PELLETS MIGHT HAVE CERTAIN NEGATIVE EFFECTS, THOUGH

There are benefits to using pellets as a long-term dosage strategy for low testosterone, but there are also downsides.

Pellets may "extrude" through the skin, or develop an infection, on rare occasions. Infection occurs in only around 0.3–0.4% of cases, and extrusion occurs in only about 0.3–1.1% of cases, therefore this is extremely uncommon.

Another surgical procedure is needed to add pellets, making it difficult to easily adjust the dosage.

Before beginning testosterone pellet therapy, it is recommended that you determine your optimal testosterone dose using an alternative method of daily testosterone delivery (such as creams or patches). Get some advice from your doctor on this.

You are a candidate for testosterone pellets after you have found an effective dose at which you are experiencing the advantages without experiencing an increase in RBC or other adverse effects.

PELLETS OF PURE TESTOSTERONE FOR FEMALES

Women are also undergoing testosterone therapy, despite the controversy surrounding it. TRT, with or without extra estrogen, has been used to treat hypoactive sexual desire problem in postmenopausal women.

As a result, people report higher levels of sexual desire, more frequent orgasms, and overall greater satisfaction.

THERE MAY ALSO BE SIGNS OF PROGRESS IN THE FOLLOWING AREAS

Lean Muscle

Bone Mass

IQ test results

Vitality of the Heart

However, providing the low-dose therapy that women require is challenging at the moment. Despite the fact that testosterone pellets have been used by women, there have been no comprehensive studies conducted to assess the dangers, particularly in regards to the emergence of malignancies.

It is also considered "off-label" to administer testosterone pellets to female patients. What this means is that a medicine with U.S. Something approved by the Food and Drug Administration (FDA) for one purpose is then used for another.

The medicine is not intended for such usage, but a doctor is free to utilize it anyway they see fit. Because the FDA oversees only the manufacturing and distribution of pharmaceuticals, and not their clinical application, this is the case. As a result, your doctor is free to write you a prescription for a medication in any way they see fit.

DISCUSS YOUR SYMPTOMS WITH YOUR DOCTOR

Have a discussion with your doctor about getting on testosterone therapy. Once you've found a dose that works with your body, you can explore the best approach that works for you.

The commitment to TRT is long-term. Testosterone pellets entail additional doctor appointments and probably more expenditure. There are drawbacks, of course, but there are also advantages, like not having to inject yourself every day and not having to worry about other people getting testosterone.

IS IT HARMFUL TO HAVE LOW TESTOSTERONE

"low T," short for low testosterone, is a prevalent ailment that affects men as they age. Normal testosterone production gradually decreases with aging. According to the Urology Care Foundation, about 20% of men in their 60s have low testosterone. This percentage jumps to 30 percent among men aged 70 and older. Around fifty percent of men in their eighties see a decline in testosterone.

TESTOSTERONE WHY MEN NEED IT

The testes of a male create the sex hormone known as testosterone. This hormone is important in the development of a boy's genitalia. Testosterone is essential for the maturation of boys' bodies into men's during puberty. It promotes facial hair growth, muscle development, and a deeper voice. Testosterone is crucial to a man's libido well into adulthood.

LOW TESTOSTERONE LEVELS CAUSE WHAT

Testosterone levels naturally decline with age. There is some evidence that a man's testosterone levels decline with age. Low testosterone levels can be brought on by more than just getting older. Damage to the testicles or exposure to cancer-fighting drugs or radiation are examples of such events. Pituitary illnesses and medications that influence the pituitary, such as steroids, are two more potential triggers.

Affects of low testosterone on sexual activity

The repercussions of low testosterone on a man's health are real and significant, particularly in terms of his sexual life. Low testosterone levels in men might make it difficult to get and maintain an erection.

They may not get erections as regularly or as hard as they used to. The urge to have sexual activity (libido) in men likewise declines when testosterone levels fall. Any or all of these may result in less frequent sexual activity. The effects on romantic partnerships might be substantial.

ALTERNATE REPERCUSSIONS OF LOW TESTOSTERONE

Having low testosterone levels impacts more than just your libido and desire to engage in sexual activity. Additionally, it may induce other symptoms. Some of the following signs may present themselves if low T is the cause

The Gain of Weight

feeling less energized than usual

decreased muscle mass and elevated fat

sad and down

struggling to focus

CONSIDERATIONS REGARDING HEALTH

The repercussions of low testosterone on the body can be devastating in the long run. For men, low levels can lead to bone weakness and even osteoporosis. People with osteoporosis are much more likely to sustain injuries.

Having low testosterone has been linked to an increased risk of dying from heart disease and other reasons, according to research published in the Journal of Clinical Endocrinology.

THE EVALUATION OF LOW TESTOSTERONE

Reduced sex drive or issues maintaining an erection are signs that a doctor visit is in need. Low testosterone can be diagnosed with a simple blood test at the doctor's office. Testosterone levels fluctuate throughout the day, so you may need to do the test more than once. Your doctor may draw blood first thing in the morning, when testosterone levels are typically at their peak.

THE PROCESS OF TREATING LOW TESTOSTERONE

Replacement therapy with testosterone may be recommended if your levels are low. The Urology Support Foundation reports that the majority of men who suffer from low testosterone apply testosterone gel to their arms and shoulders. You can also get a shot into a muscle, or you can put on a patch that slowly releases testosterone into your bloodstream. Subcutaneous pellets are another option. In addition to injectable therapy, oral replacement therapies are available. The growth of cancer can be fueled by testosterone, thus it's not recommended for men with prostate cancer to take it.

KNOWING WHEN YOU NEED THERAPY

Many pharmaceutical firms have recently begun marketing medications to treat low testosterone levels (or "low T"). A research paper released in 2011 found that the number of men over the age of 40 who used testosterone therapy increased between 2001 and 2011. If you're experiencing low testosterone symptoms, you should get tested to make sure you actually require treatment.

chapter 3

HYPOGONADISM

Hypogonadism is characterized by low or absent production of sex hormones by the gonads. Teens and adults of both sexes are vulnerable. The lack of sexual desire or libido is a symptom of this illness. Hypogonadism, also known as gonad deficit, is characterized by an absence of one or both testes.

EXPLAIN HYPOGONADISM

Hypogonadism is a condition in which the testes and ovaries produce insufficient quantities of sex hormones. The testes and ovaries are the two main components of the sex glands, often known as the gonads. Hormones secreted by both sexes play a role in regulating secondary sex characteristics such the growth of breast tissue in females and testicles in males, as well as the production of hair in the pubic region. The menstrual cycle and sperm production both depend on sex hormones.

Hypogonadism is a condition in which one or both testes are underdeveloped. When it occurs in guys, it may be referred to as low serum testosterone or andropause.

The majority of patients who receive treatment for this illness improve significantly.

EXACTLY HOW MANY DISTINCT FORMS OF HYPOGONADISM ARE THERE

Primary and central hypogonadism are the two categories of this disorder.

Hypogonadism of the primary hypothalamus

To put it simply, if you have primary hypogonadism, your gonads aren't producing enough sex hormones. Your brain is still sending signals to your gonads to make hormones, but your gonads are incapable of actually doing so.

HYPOGONADISM THAT IS CENTERED IN THE BODY

When you have central hypogonadism, the issue is on the cerebral level. The malfunctioning of your gonads is due to issues with your hypothalamus and pituitary gland.

WHY DOES HYPOGONADISM OCCUR

Primary hypogonadism has a number of root causes.

diseases caused by the body attacking itself include Addison's and hypoparathyroidism.

Turner syndrome, Klinefelter syndrome, and other genetic illnesses dangerous illnesses, most notably testicular mumps

Chronic illnesses of the liver and kidneys Having testicles that have not yet descended hemochromatosis, a condition caused by an excessive amount of absorbed iron Contamination with Radiation alteration of the genitalia.

POSSIBLE CAUSES OF CENTRAL HYPOGONADISM INCLUDE

illness of the genes, like Kalman syndrome abnormal hypothalamic development

PROBLEMS WITH THE PITUITARY GLAND

illnesses with inflammation, such as sarcoidosis, TB, and histiocytosis

OBESITY

quickly dropping pounds

Deficiencies in nutrition

injection of steroids or opioids

Surgical procedure on the brain

Contamination with Radiation

If you've sustained damage to your hypothalamus or pituitary, you may have problems controlling your emotions.

the presence of a tumor on or near the pituitary gland

EXPLAIN THE SIGNS OF HYPOGONADISM

failure to menstruate

insufficient or no breast development

the occurrence of sudden, intense heat

balding is the loss of hair from anywhere on the body.

absence of or difficulty maintaining sexual desire

milky breast secretions

MALES MAY HAVE THE FOLLOWING SYMPTOMS, AMONG OTHERS

hair thinning

decline in muscle mass

Unusual development of the breasts

penile and testicular growth retardation

ED, or impotence,

osteoporosis

absence of or difficulty maintaining sexual desire

infertility

fatigue

the occurrence of sudden, intense heat

Trouble focusing

HOW DO MEDICAL PROFESSIONALS IDENTIFY HYPOGONADISM IN A PATIENT

To ensure your sexual development is on track for your age, your doctor will do a physical examination. They may take a look at your musculature, hair, and genitalia.

TESTS FOR HORMONES

First, your doctor will likely evaluate your sex hormone levels if they suspect hypogonadism. In order to determine your follicle-stimulating hormone (FSH) and luteinizing hormone (LH) levels, a blood test will be required. Reproductive hormones are produced by the pituitary gland.

If you happen to be a female, your estrogen levels will be checked. A man's testosterone will be checked. Hormone levels are typically measured first thing in the morning. Your doctor may also request a semen analysis if you are a man and want to know how many sperm you have. A low sperm count may be an indication of hypogonadism.

In order to confirm a diagnosis and rule out potential reasons, your doctor may conduct additional blood tests.

Sex hormone production can be impacted by iron levels. Your doctor may perform a blood test to look for signs of hemochromatosis, which causes abnormally high levels of iron in the blood.

Prolactin levels are something else your doctor may want to check. Although it is more prevalent in females, prolactin is a hormone present in both sexes that encourages the growth and production of breast tissue and milk in lactating mothers.

Thyroid hormone levels are something else your doctor may look at.

Hypogonadism-like symptoms may also be brought on by thyroid issues.

EXAMINING THE IMAGE

Diagnostic imaging techniques are becoming much more widespread. With the aid of sound waves, an ultrasound can produce an image of the ovaries, allowing for a thorough examination of the reproductive system.

If your doctor suspects that you have a tumor in your pituitary gland, he or she may order an MRI or CT scan to detect it.

HYPOGONADISM IN WOMEN HOW TO TREAT IT

Treatment for women will involve a rise in levels of female sex hormones.

If you've had a hysterectomy, estrogen medication is likely to be your first line of defense. Added estrogen can be taken orally or via a transdermal patch.

If you haven't had a hysterectomy, your doctor may prescribe a combination of estrogen and progesterone to reduce your chance of developing endometrial cancer caused by having high estrogen levels. If you are taking estrogen, taking progesterone can help reduce your risk of developing endometrial cancer.

Symptoms can be specifically addressed by using alternative remedies. Reduced libido can be helped by low dosages of testosterone. Human chorionic gonadotropin injections and/or FSH tablets are used to induce ovulation in women who have problems getting pregnant or having regular periods.

HYPOGONADISM TREATMENT FOR MALES

The male sexual hormone is called testosterone. Treatment for hypogonadism in men typically entails testosterone replacement therapy.

Testosterone replacement therapy can be obtained by

Injection

Patch

gel

lozenge

Gonadotropin-releasing hormone injections may cause puberty or stimulate spermatogenesis.

HYPOGONADISM MEDICATION FOR BOTH SEXES

When a pituitary gland tumor is to blame for hypogonadism, treatment is the same for both sexes. Methods that may be used in an effort to reduce or eliminate the tumor include

radiation

medication

surgery

HOW DO THINGS LOOK DOWN THE ROAD

Hypogonadism is a long-term disorder that may require therapy for the rest of one's life unless it is caused by something that may be remedied. If you stop taking your sex hormone medication, your hormone level may drop.

Seeking aid from a therapist or support group can be beneficial before, during, and after treatment Increased levels of testosterone are beneficial.

TESTOSTERONE...WHAT IS IT

The testicles of males and the ovaries and adrenal glands of females are the primary sites of testosterone production. This hormone plays a pivotal role in shaping male physique and personality. Testosterone levels in women are significantly lower. Production of testosterone increases by a factor of 30 between puberty and early adulthood. Normal annual declines occur after early adulthood. After the age of 30, you may experience a one percent loss in physical ability.

AMONG THE MANY IMPORTANT FUNCTIONS OF TESTOSTERONE ARE

bones and muscle

Human body hair, including pubic and facial hair

deepening of the voice by physical means

passion for sex

condition of mind and existence

skill with words and brainpower

If you're worried about low testosterone, make an appointment with your doctor. Because reduced testosterone is a normal part of aging, some symptoms, such loss of muscle mass, gain in body fat, or impotence, may be indicators of something else.

If your doctor has diagnosed you with low testosterone levels (also known as hypogonadism) or recommended testosterone replacement medication for another reason, increasing your testosterone levels may be of interest to you. Increasing your testosterone levels may not have any noticeable effects if your levels are already normal. Only males with low testosterone levels have been studied for the improved benefits listed below.

WHY IS IT BENEFICIAL TO ELEVATE TESTOSTERONE LEVELS

Strong cardiovascular system and blood

The oxygen-rich blood pumped by a strong heart allows the body's muscles and organs to function at their best. Production of RBCs in the Bone Marrow is aided by Testosterone. Numerous cardiovascular problems have been related to low testosterone levels.

However, is evidence exist that testosterone replacement therapy helps with cardiovascular disease? Research findings from a Reliable Source are inconclusive. Testosterone therapy for males with heart disease resulted in modest improvements, according to early 2000s small trials. Some people even tripled their previous walking distance! One more investigation discovered that hormone therapy did nothing to alleviate angina pain but increase the diameter of healthy arteries.

Recent research involving more than 83,000 men found that men who had their testosterone levels normalized had reduced risk of heart attack by 24% and stroke by 36%.

REDUCED FAT, INCREASED MUSCLE MASS

Muscle growth is a testosterone-driven phenomenon. Muscle atrophy and increased metabolic rate both benefit from a leaner body composition. Studies have shown that treatment for low testosterone can lead to a reduction in body fat and an improvement in muscular mass and strength in males. Some males noticed an alteration in lean body mass but no improvement in strength. Combining testosterone replacement medication with weightlifting and physical activity is optimal.

HIGHER BONE DENSITY

Bone mineral density is significantly influenced by testosterone. As men age, their testosterone levels naturally decrease, which has a negative effect on bone density. There is a greater possibility of developing bone fragility and osteoporosis as a result of this. Athletes benefit from having strong bones because they provide a stable foundation for their muscles and internal organs.

As long as the dosage is high enough, testosterone therapy has been shown to promote bone density. Bone density increases in the spine and hips were observed in clinical trials evaluating testosterone's influence on bone density. Bone mineral density was observed to increase with testosterone in a separate research comparing women through andropause to men. However, it is unclear whether testosterone can aid in decreasing fracture risk.

A heightened capacity for verbal memory, visual perception, or logical analysis

According to studies, males whose total testosterone to estrogen ratio is higher also have a lower risk of developing Alzheimer's disease. Testosterone has been linked to improved cognitive functions as verbal memory and processing speed. Men aged 34 to 70 who received testosterone therapy showed enhanced spatial memory.

STRENGTHENED LIBIDO

When a man is sexually aroused and active, his testosterone levels will increase naturally. Men who have more of the hormone testosterone tend to engage in more sexual activity overall. For older men to maintain their libido and erections, they need to take in more testosterone. However, it should be noted that low testosterone levels are not always the cause of erectile dysfunction.

Research suggests that testosterone therapy can improve sexual health and function. The research also indicates that there is an upper limit to testosterone levels beyond which no further reaction is shown. Increasing testosterone levels might not improve libido in guys who don't have hypogonadism.

LIFTED SPIRITS

The quality of life decreases with declining testosterone levels. Low amounts of testosterone can cause a variety of negative emotions and behaviors, such as depression, exhaustion, and irritability. However, there is evidence from a few studies to suggest that this is applicable only to males with hypogonadism. Those males whose bodies naturally lower testosterone levels didn't show any signs of increased depression.

Replacement therapy with testosterone may have varying emotional outcomes. Source treatment for hypogonadism in men led to more happiness, less fatigue, and less irritation. In addition to its potential effectiveness as a psychiatric treatment, this method has shown promise in studies as an antidepressant.

THE HAZARDS OF TESTOSTERONE REPLACEMENT THERAPY.

Prescription testosterone therapies include gels, skin patches, and injections. Each may produce some undesirable effects in some people. It's possible for patches to cause skin irritation. Getting an intramuscular injection could affect your disposition. Do not allow anyone else to use the gel once you have tried it yourself.

These are some of the possible negative consequences of testosterone replacement therapy

worsening acne

To keep fluids in

the need to urinate more frequently

enhancement of the bust

reduced sperm count

Reduced number of sperm

aggression has escalated

In males who have had breast or prostate cancer, testosterone therapy is not recommended. The use of testosterone replacement treatment has also been linked to a worsening of sleep apnea in older adults.

ARE YOU THINKING ABOUT GETTING TESTOSTERONE INJECTIONS

If your levels are within the normal range, treatment is not necessary. Men with low testosterone levels can benefit greatly from testosterone replacement therapy. You should never get testosterone without a doctor's order. If you are concerned that your testosterone levels are too low, it is important to see a doctor. Testosterone levels can be measured using a blood test, which can also reveal other health issues.

Both medical professionals and academics are split on whether or not testosterone replacement treatment actually works. Consensus among experts suggests that studies' findings are inconsistent for most illnesses.

Optimal health and the success of testosterone therapy depend on a balanced diet and regular exercise. It is suggested to have a follow-up checkup and monitoring.

chapter 4

AGE RELATED CHANGES IN TESTOSTERONE

In both sexes, testosterone acts as a potent hormone. Among its many benefits is the capacity to moderate sexual desire, manage sperm output, build muscular mass, and boost vitality. Human hostility and competitiveness are just two behaviors that can be influenced by this.

The production of testosterone naturally declines with age. This can have a wide range of side effects, including diminished sex drive. Lowered testosterone is a normal aspect of the aging process, despite the fact that it may cause concern.

NORMAL AMOUNTS OF TESTOSTERONE

Thyroid health, protein availability, and other factors all influence what constitutes a "normal" or "healthy" level of testosterone in the blood.

To be considered normal, a man's testosterone level must be at least 300 ng/dL, as stated by the American Urological Association (AUA) in their most recent set of guidelines. In men, low testosterone is defined as a serum concentration of less than 300 ng/dL.

As a man enters adulthood, his testosterone levels rise until around age 18 or 19, and then gradually decline.

BEFORE BIRTH

When pregnant, testosterone is essential for healthy fetal growth and development.

The maturation of the male reproductive system is under its watchful eye.

One research of 60 children suggests that prenatal testosterone levels may also influence the balance of activity between the right and left hemispheres of the brain.

Fetal brain development depends on testosterone levels staying within a relatively restricted range. Intense amounts of testosterone during pregnancy have been related to autism.

EARLY ADULTHOOD TO LATE ADOLESCENCE

The peak levels of testosterone occur between puberty and early adulthood.

It is during puberty that testosterone and other androgens first manifest themselves physically in young males. When a boy transitions into manhood, he develops a deeper voice, wider shoulders, and more squared off features.

ADULTHOOD

After the age of 30, a man's testosterone levels may drop by about 1% annually.

The ovaries are the primary site of testosterone production in premenopausal females. After menopause, which typically begins between the ages of 45 and 55, levels drop.

MALE HORMONE DEFICIENCY SYMPTOMS

The quantity of testosterone in your system can be determined with a blood test.

However, low testosterone levels can also be a result of medical disorders present from birth. Having a low testosterone level is possible if your testicles or ovaries, the organs responsible for producing the hormone, have been damaged by an illness.

Aging can cause a decline in levels. On the other hand, America has its own problems. The FDA recommends against testosterone replacement treatment (TRT) for low levels due to aging.

ALTERATIONS IN SEXUAL FUNCTION CAN OCCUR WHEN TESTOSTERONE LEVELS ARE TOO LOW

low libido, or lack of sexual desire

reduced number of 'acts of virility'

impotence

Impairment of the ability to get or keep an erection (ED)

infertility

ADDITIONAL SYMPTOMS OF LOW TESTOSTERONE LEVELS ARE

alterations in the way one sleeps

Trouble focusing

failure to inspire action

depleted muscular mass and power

loss of bone mass

the condition of having unusually big male breasts

depression

fatigue

You should get checked for low testosterone levels if you suspect you may have them.

RELATIONSHIPS BETWEEN FEMALES AND TESTOSTERONE

While testosterone is primarily a masculine hormone, it is essential for both sexes. Less testosterone is present in females than males.

After a woman reaches menopause, her estrogen levels begin to decline. This could cause a little increase in her levels of androgens (male hormones). Testosterone levels can also be impacted by diseases like polycystic ovary syndrome (PCOS).

IN WOMEN, HIGH LEVELS OF TESTOSTERONE IN THE BLOOD CAN LEAD TO

hair loss on the scalp

acne

period disruptions or absences

development of a beard or mustache

infertility

Infertility is another potential outcome of low testosterone in women, following on the heels of brittle bones and a lack of interest in sexual activity.

DIAGNOSIS AND TESTING

Low testosterone is best diagnosed with a trip to the doctor for a physical and some blood work.

Your doctor will evaluate your overall health and sexual maturity. It's recommended to take the blood sample before 10 a.m., as testosterone levels tend to be highest first thing in the morning. with younger males. Up until 2 pm, men over 45 can take the test. while yet obtaining reliable outcomes.

Risks linked with the blood test are low but may include bleeding, discomfort at the injection site, or infection.

IMPLICATIONS OF EXCESSIVE OR INSUFFICIENT TESTOSTERONE

Signs of low testosterone can just be part of becoming older, but they could also indicate something more serious. Here are some of them

reaction to medication

Disturbances of the Thyroid Gland

depression

heavy drinking

Lowered testosterone levels may result from a number of factors, including but not limited to

testicular or ovarian cancer

ineffectiveness of the testicles

low gonad hormone production, often known as hypogonadism.

Immature sexual development

condition that lasts a long time, as diabetes or kidney disease

extreme fatness

radiation treatment or chemotherapy

Use of Opioids

congenital defects that can be traced back to a faulty gene, like Klinefelter syndrome

High amounts of testosterone could result from

PCOS

CAH is a condition that affects females from birth.

cancers of the adrenal glands or gonads

Takeaway

your doctor may recommend trt if he finds that your testosterone levels are too low. forms of testosterone include

the administration of a shot

a Band-Aid

Topical gel for the skin

gel inserted into the nasal passages

pellets that are surgically inserted under he skin

A number of medicines are available for the treatment of elevated testosterone levels in women.

methods of contraception administered orally

SPIRONOLACTONE
ALDACTONE

Worry over decreased testosterone levels is only natural. This, however, is to be expected as a natural consequence of becoming older. If you're concerned or exhibiting unusual symptoms, it's important to schedule an appointment with your doctor.

chapter 5

METHODS THAT HAVE BEEN PROVEN TO BOOST TESTOSTERONE NATURALLY

The hormone testosterone affects everything from sexual performance to the likelihood of contracting certain diseases. Discover how natural methods, like weightlifting, can help you raise your testosterone levels.

The primary androgenic hormone in men is testosterone. Some trace levels are also present in people who were assigned female at birth.

The testicles and ovaries are the primary organs responsible for producing this steroid hormone. Small amounts are also produced by the adrenal glands.

GETTING A GOOD NIGHT'S REST

Lack of sleep has been linked to decreased levels of testosterone and other essential hormones and substances.

Men who don't get enough sleep may see a decline in testosterone, according to research from the University of Source.

After 10 healthy males, all approximately 24 years old, spent 1 week sleeping 8 hours each night at home, they spent the following 11 nights in a laboratory. For the first three nights, they got a full night's sleep of 10 hours, but for the next eight, they were forced to limit their sleep to just five. On the night before the 10-hour sleep restriction, doctors monitored their blood every 15 to 30 minutes.

Sleep deprivation for just one week was found to reduce daytime testosterone levels by up to 15%, according to the study. In contrast, testosterone levels gradually decline with age at a rate of only 2% each year in healthy adults.

Making sleep a priority may help sustain testosterone levels. Sleeping for at least seven or eight hours a night should be a daily goal. Sleep difficulties should be discussed with a medical professional.

EATING WELL REQUIRES DISCIPLINE

Eating healthily has long been known to be critical for keeping testosterone levels and general health at optimal levels. One report Source suggests that low levels of testosterone and being overweight can both contribute to a number of inflammatory diseases and decreased brain function.

Hormone levels were shown to be disturbed by excessive eating and yo-yo dieting. People who engage in strenuous physical activity, such as sports, are more likely to notice this effect.

A diet that is high in whole foods and provides a good balance of fats, carbs, and proteins is optimal. Maintaining a healthy hormonal balance is just one more benefit of eating a balanced and nutritious diet that can help you live a long and happy life.

LOSE WEIGHT

The testosterone levels of overweight males have been demonstrated to be lower. One study published in Clinical Endocrinology Source found that testosterone levels were up to 50% lower in overweight men aged 14-20 compared to lean men of the same age.

KEEP MOVING AROUND

Researchers found that the more physically active a person was, the higher their testosterone levels were.

According to the source, raising testosterone levels with increased physical activity is preferable to doing so through weight loss alone.

Extreme activity, though, can reduce testosterone levels, so moderation is key.

Indeed, the same study suggested that low testosterone levels could be a problem for long-distance runners. The study's authors argued that low levels of energy and poor nutrition could be to blame.

CONQUERING STRESS

Prolonged or persistent stress is harmful and can cause a variety of health problems.

Cortisol, which is increased by stress, regulates many bodily functions, from the immune system to energy expenditure.

High levels of cortisol suppress testosterone. According to the study cited, male testosterone levels fluctuate erratically when men experience stress.

Over the course of two months preceding their final exams, 58 male and female medical students completed questionnaires and provided saliva samples while under exam stress.

Salivary testosterone levels increased significantly in the men in the study when they were stressed about exams, but they fell significantly in the women.

Researchers speculate that disparities between the sexes can be explained by the fact that male study participants had a more aggressive, emotionally inhibited, and ruminative stress reaction.

FOOD ADDITIVES AND VITAMINS

Vitamin D supplementation has been linked to improved testosterone levels and the correction of vitamin D deficiency, according to research published in the Journal of Hormone Source.

Vitamin D levels can also be maintained by exposing oneself to sunlight for at least 15 minutes every day. Salmon and other fatty fishes, as well as fortified milk and cereal products, are good dietary sources of vitamin D.

DHEA dehydroepiandrosterone is a hormone involved in the creation of testosterone and other hormones that regulate body fat. DHEA levels, like testosterone levels, decline with age. In one experiment, older males were given DHEA supplements. Positive changes in body composition, albeit slight, were observed after taking the supplements, according to the study.

Eating fish and flaxseed, which are both high in healthy fats, may improve your body's ability to use the DHEA it creates.

If a magnesium deficit is to blame for low testosterone levels, using magnesium supplements can help restore normal levels.

Taking supplements for at least a month has been shown to have the potential to raise testosterone levels in all persons, according to a study published in the journal Biological Trace Element Research. According to the study, those who exercise regularly see a greater rise in testosterone than their less active counterparts.

As with magnesium, zinc insufficiency may contribute to a reduction in testosterone. A 2 study with reliable results found that supplementing with zinc for 4 weeks prevented a drop in testosterone levels in sedentary men who exercised.

Magnesium and zinc deficiencies, on the other hand, can be treated with food. Magnesium-rich foods include whole grains and dark leafy greens. Dark greens, flax seeds, and pumpkin seeds are other good sources of zinc.

Creatine is widely known to reliably and modestly raise testosterone levels. In a study conducted in 2006, Source found that after supplementing with creatine for at least 10 weeks, college football players saw increased levels of testosterone. The protein-rich salmon, tuna, and beef all contain creatine naturally.

PRESCRIPTION DRUG EVALUATION

While there are many problems that can be helped by using prescription drugs, low testosterone is a common side effect.

One research source suggests that statins, a kind of cholesterol-lowering drugs, may also function in part by decreasing testosterone levels in the body.

Anyone who feels low testosterone is linked to prescribed drugs should bring these concerns to their doctor's notice.

STAY AWAY FROM ALCOHOL AND DRUGS

Low testosterone has been connected to substance abuse.

The National Institutes of Health reports that drinking alcohol can disrupt the function of the testes and other reproductive organs in men.

Further, alcohol's effects on the body, such as producing hormonal reactions and cell damage, can lead to reduced testosterone levels.

POSSIBLE FOODS TO INCREASE TESTOSTERONE

Low testosterone is common as people become older, but it can also be caused by things like certain drugs, high body fat, and certain health disorders .

Hypogonadism, often known as low T or low testosterone, is diagnosed when serum testosterone levels are below 300 ng/dL. Replacement therapy with testosterone is a medical option for men with low testosterone.

Hypogonadism affects a large percentage of the population. Approximately 40% of males over 45 and 50% of men over 80 are diagnosed as hypogonadal.

Keeping your testosterone levels at their peak requires a commitment to a healthful lifestyle, which includes eating well. Diets heavy in ultra-processed foods and low in nutrient-dense foods have been linked in some research to lower testosterone levels.

If your doctor tells you that your testosterone levels are low, do what they say. In addition, your diet could benefit from an increase in the types of food that are high in nutrients that are necessary for keeping your testosterone levels normal.

SPECIES OF FISH HIGH IN SATURATED FAT

Vitamin D, zinc, and omega-3 fatty acids are all essential for proper hormonal function, and fatty fish like salmon and sardines are a great source of all three.

While studies have shown that consuming high-fat foods like fried foods might cause low testosterone levels in some men, studies have also shown that low-fat diets can be harmful for testosterone levels.

The testosterone levels of men who followed low-fat diets were shown to be lower than those who followed higher-fat diets, according to a meta-analysis of six research .

Researchers did say that more high quality studies are needed to completely grasp this association though .

Regardless, it's likely good for your health to include hormonal health to add healthy sources of fat like fatty fish to your diet.

In addition, the zinc, vitamin D, and protein found in fatty fish are all essential components for normal testosterone function.

Scientists have shown that testosterone levels are often lower in men with low vitamin D levels. Because vitamin D is crucial to men's reproductive health, this is the case.

THOSE DARK LEAFY GREENS

Magnesium, a mineral vital for maintaining optimum testosterone levels, especially in older men, is abundant in dark, leafy greens.

Some researchers believe that because magnesium lowers oxidative stress, its presence in the body causes more testosterone bioactivity. A state of oxidative stress occurs when the body's antioxidant defenses are overwhelmed by the body's free radicals.

Nutrients that fight oxidative stress and inflammation may help keep testosterone levels stable.

An older study including males aged 65 and over indicated that those whose blood magnesium levels were greater also had higher testosterone levels.

Furthermore, a study in Taiwanese men connected low testosterone levels to a lack of consumption of leafy green vegetables.

Therefore, consuming more vegetables rich in magnesium, such as spinach, kale, and collard greens, may aid in maintaining normal testosterone levels.

CHOCOLATIER WARES

Magnesium and flavonoid antioxidants, found in abundance in cocoa products like cocoa powder and cacao nibs, are crucial for testosterone production.

Flavonoids are chemicals found in plants that have strong antioxidant and anti-inflammatory actions.

Cocoa flavonoids, such as quercetin and apigenin, have been linked to an increase in testosterone production by a kind of testicular cell called a Leydig cell.

The best cocoa products to buy are those that have either no added sugar or very little added sugar. If you're looking for a healthy alternative to regular chocolate, try cocoa powder, cacao nibs, or low sugar dark chocolate.

AVOCADOS

Healthy fat, such that found in avocados, plays a role in maintaining balanced hormones. Additionally, avocados are rich in magnesium and a mineral called boron, both of which may improve testosterone levels.

Boron, a common trace mineral, has been shown to affect testosterone metabolism and provide protection against testosterone breakdown in the body.

The results of investigations on the effects of supplemental high amounts of boron on testosterone levels are inconsistent. The effects of boron supplements on testosterone levels need further study.

There is no consensus on whether or whether using boron supplements will boost testosterone levels, but including foods like avocados in your diet can help you get the mineral you need may help keep your testosterone levels stable.

EGGS

Egg yolks are an excellent source of protein, healthy fat, and the antioxidant mineral selenium.

Some in vitro and animal research suggests that selenium can stimulate the expression of specific genes and the corresponding pathways, hence increasing testosterone synthesis.

Testosterone levels are also observed to be higher in those with adequate blood selenium levels, according to several research in both humans and animals.

To make firm conclusions on selenium's impact on testosterone, however, further research is needed, particularly in humans.

Unless you have an egg allergy, you should incorporate eggs into your diet if you aren't currently doing so. Don't forget that the yolks of eggs are where most of the beneficial nutrients are found, making whole eggs far more beneficial than just the whites.

POMEGRANATES, CHERRIES, AND BERRIES

Flavonoid antioxidants, which are abundant in berries, cherries, and pomegranates, have been shown to protect testosterone-producing cells from harm and boost testosterone production.

Supplementation with pomegranate juice raised testosterone levels and protected the Leydig cells (responsible for testosterone production) from damage, according to an older study in rats.

Whether or whether pomegranates or their juice have an effect on testosterone levels requires more human research.

Anti-inflammatory foods including pomegranates, berries, and cherries may protect against the testosterone-lowering effects of obesity-induced inflammation.

Hormonal health may benefit from a diet rich in antioxidant-rich foods like these fruits.

SHELLFISH

Oysters, clams, and other shellfish may help keep testosterone levels at a healthy level since they are rich in zinc, selenium, and omega-3 fatty acids.

A lack of zinc, which plays an essential role in reproductive health, can lead to hypogonadism.

It has also been shown that high-dose zinc tablets can help males who suffer from hypogonadism. Even yet, zinc supplements are not generally advocated as a one-size-fits-all solution for hypogonadism.

But eating foods rich in minerals like zinc, selenium, and omega-3 fats, which are all necessary for maintaining healthy testosterone levels, may boost hormonal health.

chapter 6

FOODS THAT ARE LOW IN TESTOSTERONE

There is evidence that consuming soy, dairy, and certain fats can reduce testosterone levels.

Normalizing one's weight and engaging in regular physical activity are two natural ways to boost testosterone levels.

A person's diet can have an effect on more than just their waistline. The nutrients in food provide energy for the body's cells and may have an effect on hormones like testosterone.

Some foods, when consumed in large quantities, may disrupt the body's hormonal balance or make it more challenging for the body to use hormones properly.

POTENTIALLY LOW TESTOSTERONE LOWERING FOODS

Testosterone levels may drop as a result of consuming soy or drinking alcohol.

Testosterone is an important sex hormone. Testosterone is an essential hormone for both males and women. Gains in strength, bone density, and hair density are all aided by testosterone, and the hormone also affects ovulation and pregnancy.

Normal testosterone levels are maintained through the body's efficient regulation of hormones.

However, the hormonal balance can be disrupted by eating certain foods. For those who are concerned about their testosterone levels, avoiding the following meals may be a good idea.

SOYBEANS AND THEIR BY PRODUCTS

Phytoestrogens can be found in soy products such tofu, edamame, and soy protein isolates. These chemicals mimic the action of endogenous estrogen because of their structural similarities.

Despite extensive investigation, researchers acknowledge that some questions remain about soy, according to a study published in Medical Science Source.

According to the report, researchers have been unable to establish a link between soy consumption and changes in serum testosterone or estrogen levels. However, another study found that if men quit consuming soy, their breast soreness and hormone levels reverted to normal.

According to the study's authors, phytoestrogens in soy may have physiological effects without causing the usual rise in estrogen levels.

More rigorous studies in both sexes are needed to determine the full range of soy's physiological effects.

DAIRY GOODS

It's possible that many men who want to boost their testosterone levels would rather not consume dairy products. Perhaps this is due to the presence of synthetic or natural hormones in some varieties of cow's milk, which may have an effect on testosterone levels.

The use of soy in animal feed has been linked to elevated estrogen levels in milk produced from cows.

ALCOHOL

If you're worried about your testosterone levels, you might want to cut back or stop drinking entirely. Perhaps this is truer of men than women.

While preliminary research suggests that drinking alcohol may have a positive effect on testosterone levels in males, more extensive studies are needed to draw firm conclusions. One study published in Current Drug Trusted Source found that men who drink heavily or regularly for extended periods of time had lower levels of the male hormone testosterone.

According to the report, female testosterone levels rise after drinking alcohol.

MINT

Men's testosterone levels might be lowered by mint, according to the research.

While a cup of peppermint or spearmint tea could help you relax, the menthol in mint might actually lower your testosterone.

A study published in Advanced Pharmaceutical Source reports that essential oil of spearmint was used to treat polycystic ovary syndrome (PCOS) in female rats. Spearmint essential oil was found to decrease testosterone levels in these rats.

Mint has been shown to reduce testosterone levels in women with polycystic ovary syndrome, according to a review published in BMC Complementary & Alternative Source. But there isn't nearly enough high-quality research to support the herb's general effect.

Most studies on this area involve either female subjects or animal models. It is important to study the effects of mint in both sexes in future studies.

DESSERTS BAKED GOODS AND BREAD

One study found that men in Taiwan with a diet heavy in sweets and baked goods had significantly lower total testosterone levels than those with a more savory diet. Other contributors included a diet low in green vegetables and rich in dairy and restaurant meals.

The men in the report also had lower muscle mass and higher body fat percentages.

GENUS GLYCYRRHIZA

An article published in Integrative Medicine Research Source reports that licorice root can lower testosterone levels in otherwise healthy women before and during their periods. Testosterone levels can be lowered by taking licorice, according to animal research.

To gain a more complete picture of licorice's actions, future research should ideally examine the herb's impacts on both sexes.

FATS THAT ARE GOOD FOR YOU

A person's testosterone levels and functionality may also be affected by the sort of fat they eat. Hormone levels and testicular health were studied in relation to the eating habits of young, healthy males in a study published in the Asian Journal of Andrology Source.

They found that consuming trans fats was associated with reduced testosterone levels. Researchers also discovered that an excess of omega-6 fatty acids diminished testicular growth and function.

On the other hand, getting enough polyunsaturated omega-3 fatty acids may help your testicles grow and work better. Although more research is needed to validate these results, men concerned about their testosterone levels may choose to reduce their intake of trans fats and increase their intake of omega-6 fats.

Chapter 7

TESTOSTERONE BOOSTING SUPPLEMENTS

Your testosterone levels can be boosted by taking one of several supplements. The findings are inconclusive. The following are examples of such aids

THE D-ASPARTIC ACID

The amino acid D-aspartic acid occurs in the human body. Follicle-stimulating hormone and luteinizing hormone levels may be raised, according to a recent study. These two factors may work together to increase testosterone production in the body.

A later study, however, found that 3 grams of D-aspartic acid had no effect on testosterone levels. The levels were really decreased by taking 6 grams.

ZINC

The element zinc is crucial to proper bodily function. Low levels of testosterone have been linked to zinc insufficiency. The testes may produce more testosterone if zinc levels are high. In theory, zinc supplementation over a long period of time could raise testosterone levels.

MAGNESIUM

Supplemental magnesium has been demonstrated to raise both free and total testosterone. Potential beneficiaries include both couch potatoes and athletes. Remember that persons whose testosterone levels naturally increased during exercise experienced much greater increases.

VITAMIN D

When skin is exposed to sunshine, the body makes its own Vitamin D. However, vitamin D deficiency is possible in persons who don't get enough sunlight. Testosterone levels were found to be 20% higher in the group that took 3300 IU of vitamin D daily compared to the control group.

WHICH HERBS HELP SUPPORT TESTOSTERONE THE MOST

The male hormone testosterone is crucial for sexual performance. It aids in the development of typically male traits and the upkeep of adult male health. A man's libido, physical prowess, mental state, and outlook can all suffer from low testosterone levels. Roughly five million men in the United States have low testosterone levels but aren't being treated for it. Now that there are so many effective methods of increasing testosterone levels, men who have Low T no longer have to accept their condition.

Low testosterone levels in males can be brought back up to normal with the use of testosterone replacement therapy and testosterone-boosting items, such as some natural vitamins and herbs.

HERBS THAT BOOST MEN'S TESTOSTERONE NATURALLY

It is possible to increase testosterone production with the help of herbs. Numerous herbal formulae, including ginseng, yohimbe, saw palmetto, nettles, maca root, catauba, Tribulus terrestris, and pycnogenol, are used to enhance testosterone levels in men. These formulas also increase a man's energy, stamina, and endurance, as well as his sexual desire.

Athletes, weightlifters, and bodybuilders often sing the praises of natural testosterone boosters for their capacity to help them bulk up, slim down, get defined, and shed unwanted fat. Talk to your hormone doctor before starting Low T treatment if testosterone supplements are part of your healthcare regimen. This will allow your doctor to correctly incorporate them into your HRT program.

GINSENG

For thousands of years, ginseng has been used as part of traditional Chinese medicine. Healers of all stripes and from all corners of the globe now turn to ginseng for its myriad therapeutic benefits. Ginseng is well-known for its stimulating effects, including increased energy and decreased stress and fatigue, and for its capacity to improve sexual performance. A number of ginseng varieties are available, and they're all popular. In the United States, ginseng is grown commercially in ginseng farms, specifically in the country's mountainous regions. The dried roots of Asian ginseng are then made into extracts, capsules, pills, and teas. Topical therapies can also be administered with external preparations. The root's active chemical ingredients help with things like erectile dysfunction, hepatitis C, and increasing testosterone levels and stamina.

YOHIMBE

It is the bark of the yohimbe tree in western Africa that is used to make the herb yohimbe. The plant can be found in tablets, pills, and teas, and it is used to treat sexual dysfunction, as an aphrodisiac, to boost testosterone, to construct muscle, to calm anxiety, and to aid in weight loss. Yohimbe, when applied topically, has an anesthetic effect. Yohimbe has psychedelic effects when smoked. Its use is not without risk, as it has been linked to anxiety, hypertension, headaches, and sleeplessness.

THE TERMITE TRIBULUS

Tribulus terrestris has a long history of usage as an aphrodisiac and general health tonic in Ayurvedic medicine. Luteinizing Hormones (LH) enhance testosterone production, and tribulus has been shown to raise LH levels. In traditional medicine, the plant was used to treat a variety of ailments across Europe, including headaches, mental disorders, constipation, and erectile dysfunction. The plant has been used to treat high blood pressure, high cholesterol, liver disease, and cardiovascular disease in numerous cultures. Because of its historical and current use in increasing testosterone and muscle mass, the plant is often used by athletes and bodybuilders. Goat head, or caltrop, is a plant that tends to pop up in odd places like along the side of the road or in otherwise desolate arcas. It grows in clusters and produces thorny green clumps at the tips of its many stems. Southern Asia, Europe, Africa, Australia, and the United States are all home to this plant.

MACA ROOT

Cayenne Pepper, Stinging Nettles, Catauba, Ginger, Carao, Epimedium (also known as horny goat), and Catauba Leaf

Free testosterone levels can be increased in a novel way by using a highly concentrated extract from the nettle root. Components of stinging nettle root have been identified by European researchers to compete with testosterone for binding to SHBG, hence decreasing SHBG's binding of free testosterone.

Catauba, a tree native to the Amazonian jungle, is known to increase testosterone levels in men.

In order to increase testosterone levels, maca root includes a substance known as p-methoxybenzyl isothiocyanate.

The testosterone-boosting properties of ginger also aid in increasing blood flow to the vaginal area.

Horny goat weed, also known as epimedium, is taken to combat weariness and increase testosterone levels.

The Costa Rican fruit caao is used as a treatment for anemia, and it also boosts testosterone levels in the body.

Cayenne Fruit increases testosterone and aids fat burning by bolstering the cardiovascular system, blood vessels, and nervous system.

L-ARGININE AN AMINO ACID THAT INCREASES TESTOSTERONE

L-Arginine improves erection strength by raising testosterone and enhancing nitric oxide synthesis, which in turn promotes muscle growth and increases blood flow to erectile tissue in the penis by relaxing blood vessel walls.

TESTOSTERONE LEVELS CAN BE INCREASED BY CONSUMING ZINC AND SELENIUM

Zinc aids in normalizing estrogen levels, allowing the body to put more of its attention on making effective use of testosterone. Zinc dosages in the 15–25 mg per day range are recommended as daily supplements. As a dietary supplement, selenium can help increase testosterone levels.

BOOSTING TESTOSTERONE THROUGH LOWERING SHBG

There are a number of herbs that increase testosterone levels, and others that stimulate the genitalia by bringing more blood to the penis. To prevent testosterone from being bound up and used by the body, some people lower SHBG levels. Unlike with increases in total testosterone, the potential negative side effects of boosting free testosterone through reducing SHBG are avoided. While a man's total testosterone level will remain unchanged, his body's ability to use that hormone will increase.

The presence of Sex Hormone Binding Globulin is associated with low mood, low libido, high risk for cardiovascular disease, and poor muscle tone.

In particular, Avenacosides can be found in the herb Avena Sativa (Oat Straw Extract). Similarly, Urtica dioica, sometimes known as stinging nettles, has been proven to decrease both SHBG and prolactin, a hormone produced primarily in females. The Amazon rainforest is the natural habitat of the herb Ptychopetalum. Muira Puama, which translates to "potency wood," is the indigenous name for the genus. Sixty-two percent of males who took Muira Puama extract claimed an increase in sex drive, while fifty-one percent of participants in a 1990 study by Jacques Waynsberg at the Institute of

Sexology in Paris reported an increase in their capacity to have an erection.

The female hormones prolactin and estrogen can be lowered with the help of certain medicines. The herb Mucuna Puriens (velvet bean) reduces prolactin levels in women whose testosterone levels have dropped because it boosts the brain's supply of L-dopa, which is converted to dopamine. Luteinizing hormone (LH) and testosterone levels are both boosted by Mucuna puriens, but prolactin levels are lowered. Estrogen is crucial for men since it aids in sperm creation, bone preservation, adipose tissue support, and cognitive function. While men do require a trace amount of estrogen to support these vital body activities, there are a number of reasons why men may develop estrogen excesses. One is that aromatase, an enzyme present in most cellular membranes, converts testosterone into estrogen. A man's aromatase enzyme production will increase along with his estrogen levels if he has a larger body fat percentage. A man's testosterone levels will naturally drop if his estrogen levels are elevated. Therefore, lowering overall body fat and estrogen levels is critical for protecting high testosterone levels.

If your doctor prescribes a Testosterone Replacement Therapy program, lowering SHBG to release bound testosterone is a great way to complement the therapy.

chapter 8

THE EFFECTS OF ALCOHOL ON TESTOSTERONE

Drinking too much alcohol is bad for your health in practically every way. It's also important for your hormones to be healthy.

Excessive alcohol use is associated with temporary and permanent alterations in testosterone levels, among other hormones.

The male sex hormone testosterone is the most important one. It's necessary for the development of muscle and bone in boys and men, as well as for the production of sperm.

Even while this article focuses on testosterone in men's health, women also produce a little amount of testosterone in their ovaries. Decreased amounts of testosterone in women can contribute to low sex drive and fragile bones.

If you want to know how drinking affects your testosterone levels, read on.

THE EFFECTS OF ALCOHOL ON TESTOSTERONE

The testes, anterior pituitary gland, and hypothalamus all have a role in the generation of testosterone in men.

Your hypothalamus releases a hormone called gonadotropin-releasing hormone (GnRH), which works on your anterior pituitary gland.

Afterward, your anterior pituitary gland secretes luteinizing hormone (LH) and follicle-stimulating hormone (FSH).

Testosterone is produced by the testes in response to luteinizing hormone (LH) and follicle-stimulating hormone (FSH).

Alcohol can affect testosterone production by interacting with all three glands.

Alcohol's long-term impact on testosterone

Poor testicular function is more common in heavy drinkers than to moderate drinkers.

Typically, a person is considered to have a heavy drinking problem if they consume more than 15 drinks per week (for men) or 8 drinks per week (for women).

WHEN MEN DRINK EXCESSIVELY, THEY INCREASE THEIR RISK OF EXPERIENCING

low circulating testosterone

a lack of sexual desire

It is believed that the cells in your testes called Leydig cells can be damaged by drinking alcohol on a regular basis. LH, FSH, and GnRH secretion could be impacted by alcohol consumption.

Consuming alcohol in moderation does not appear to negatively affect fertility or testosterone levels in men.

Moderate alcohol consumption is commonly described as no more than one drink for women or two drinks for males in a single day.

ALCOHOL'S SHORT TERM IMPACT ON TESTOSTERONE

Acute alcohol consumption is hypothesized to temporarily limit testosterone release via influencing the hypothalamus and pituitary gland.

Testosterone levels can begin to plummet as soon as 30 minutes after drinking, according to the cited study.

One study Source examined testosterone levels in alcoholic and nonalcoholic males by giving the former the equivalent of one pint of whiskey every day for 30 days.

By the end of the month, the testosterone levels of the healthy men had dropped to the same level as those of the alcoholic males.

WHAT HAPPENS TO YOUR SPERM WHEN YOU DRINK

The Sertoli cells in your testes are negatively affected by alcohol. The development of mature sperm relies on the presence of these cells.

Spermatogenesis refers to the process by which sperm develop. Testosterone and follicle stimulating hormone both contribute to spermatogenesis.

If these hormones aren't balanced, spermatogenesis can be stopped in its tracks. A low number of sperm in the semen is a possible outcome of spermatogenic arrest, which is the disruption of normal sperm development.

In comparison to sober men, heavy drinkers have a 50% higher incidence of spermatogenic arrest.

They also discovered that regular drinkers' testicles were smaller than those of nondrinkers.

Heavy drinking may reduce semen volume and alter sperm shape, according to 2017 research Source involving 16,395 healthy men. Light to moderate drinking had no discernible influence on either variable.

Research Source involving 8,344 healthy males from Europe and the United States found the same thing about moderate alcohol use and the quality of sperm.

It's general knowledge that pregnant women shouldn't drink, but new evidence reveals that fathers who imbibe heavily prior to conception may also increase their child's risk of being born with a disability.

www.ingramcontent.com/pod-product-compliance
Lightning Source LLC
Chambersburg PA
CBHW071036250726
48653CB00005B/1859